Understanding
Irritable Bowel Syndrome

Kirsten Tillisch, MD

Kieran J. Moriarty, MD, CBE

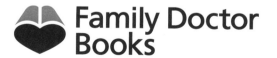

Family Doctor Books

IMPORTANT

This book is intended not as a substitute for personal medical advice but as a supplement to that advice for the patient who wishes to understand more about his or her condition.

Before taking any form of treatment
YOU SHOULD ALWAYS CONSULT YOUR MEDICAL PRACTITIONER.

In particular (without limit) you should note that advances in medical science occur rapidly and some information about drugs and treatment contained in this booklet may very soon be out of date.

© Family Doctor Publications 2006

ISBN 10: 1-4285-0005-7
ISBN 13: 978-1-4285-0005-1

Contents

About the authors

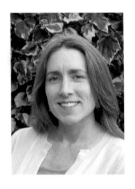

Dr. Kirsten Tillisch is a gastroenterologist specializing in the treatment of functional gastrointestinal disorders at the Center for Neurovisceral Sciences and Women's Health at UCLA. Her research interests include investigation of the brain-gut axis, the autonomic nervous system, and sex-differences in IBS.

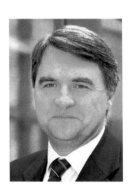

Dr. Kieran J. Moriarty, CBE is a consultant physician and gastroenterologist. He has wide experience in the treatment of patients with gastrointestinal disorders. His research interests include abdominal pain, alcohol-related problems, IBS, and bowel disorders. In 2002, he was awarded the British order of CBE for services to medicine.

Introduction

What is irritable bowel syndrome?

Irritable bowel syndrome (IBS) is one of the most common gastrointestinal disorders, but it is puzzling for those who have it and for the doctors who treat it. Unlike disorders such as stomach ulcers or arthritis, there is no laboratory test, X-ray, scan, or endoscopic investigation that can show whether or not you have IBS.

There is no clear-cut cure for the disorder. Various kinds of treatment can relieve the symptoms, however, and, with the right kind of support from your doctor, you can learn to live with it.

IBS is a syndrome, a collection of symptoms with similar features that occur together in a pattern that your doctor can recognize. In typical cases, there is rarely any doubt about the diagnosis, although you may have symptoms in any part of your gastrointestinal tract, which stretches from the esophagus to the rectum.

What are the main symptoms?

The term "irritable" is used to describe the reaction of the muscles in the intestine, which respond to stress or eating by abnormal contractions. These may result in various combinations of the three main symptoms:

- abdominal pain
- diarrhea
- constipation.

These symptoms are often worrying. However, if you have been told that you have IBS, you can take some comfort from the information that the disorder does not increase your chance of developing long-term serious conditions such as cancer or ulcerative colitis. Also, there is no evidence that people with IBS have a shorter life expectancy.

What will I find in this book?

The first five chapters of this book describe the structure and workings of the gastrointestinal tract. They explain the symptoms of IBS and how it is recognized. They also cover what is known about its causes and how common it is in people from different ethnic groups in countries around the world.

Later chapters deal with common symptoms such as constipation and diarrhea. They explain how these apparently opposite problems can be part of the same syndrome. These chapters also describe the various approaches to treatment that may be tried and how these can help. There is also practical advice on self-help measures that you may try.

The final chapters of the book discuss how people with IBS can learn to live with the disorder, and get support from a sympathetic doctor. The more that you understand about IBS and the reasons for your symptoms, the better you will be able to cope with them. We hope that this book will help you to do just that.

How common is IBS?

Irritable bowel syndrome affects around one in five adults in the industrialized countries. Even more people have at least one of its symptoms. A study performed in the United States found that, in one year, as many as 70 percent of the general population had problems associated with abnormal bowel function, such as abdominal pain, constipation, or diarrhea. IBS occurs in about 15 percent of the U.S. population.

Three-quarters of people with symptoms of IBS do not consult a doctor, and yet as many as half the people seen by a gastroenterologist (a doctor specializing in disorders of the gastrointestinal system) find that it is the cause of their problems. Evidence suggests that many of the people with IBS seen in clinics also have symptoms of depression or anxiety.

The cost of IBS to patients and to society is enormous. Average work days missed per year in the U.S. were 14.8, as compared with 8.7 in those without the symptoms of IBS. Indeed, IBS ranks close to the common cold as a leading cause for absenteeism from work as a result of illness. In the United Kingdom, around eight million people have IBS. On average, each of them took 17 days off work a year, equivalent to a cost of more than 900 million dollars.

Most surveys show that symptoms of IBS are more common in women, and women consult their doctors about these symptoms more often than men. About half of those with IBS develop symptoms before the age of 35. Forty percent of people with the condition are aged 35 through 50 years.

There is a tendency for symptoms to occur less frequently as a person ages, though some people experience them for the first time later in life. Doctors tend to be more cautious about diagnosing IBS in people who develop symptoms after age 50. They will usually do so only after excluding other diseases of the gut.

KEY POINTS

■ IBS is a syndrome, not a disease, affecting about 20 percent of adults in industrialized countries

■ Doctors see twice as many women as men with the condition

■ IBS has a major social impact, leading to frequent days off work and restriction of social activities

The gastrointestinal tract

What is the gastrointestinal tract?

The gastrointestinal tract is a long passageway that connects the mouth with the anus. Digestion starts in the mouth, where food mixes with salivary enzymes. When you swallow, food is propelled down the esophagus into the stomach. In the stomach, it is broken down by the powerful digestive enzymes and the acid found in gastric juices.

From the stomach, food passes into the small intestine (duodenum, jejunum, and ileum), where juices from the pancreas and gallbladder continue the digestive process. It is here that most of the nutrients are absorbed from food. This happens as the intestinal contents are moved along by peristalsis (movement caused by alternating muscle contraction and relaxation).

Undigested waste (feces) then moves into the large intestine (the colon). In the first part of the colon, muscle contractions slowly move it along toward the rectum while excess water is removed. Just before

The gastrointestinal tract and the digestive process

Food must be broken down so that the body can absorb the nutrients. Undigested material and waste are expelled.

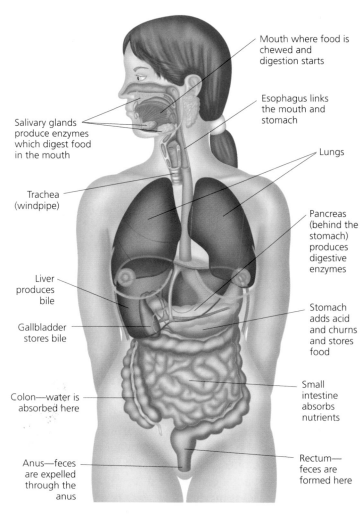

Mouth where food is chewed and digestion starts

Esophagus links the mouth and stomach

Salivary glands produce enzymes which digest food in the mouth

Lungs

Trachea (windpipe)

Pancreas (behind the stomach) produces digestive enzymes

Liver produces bile

Stomach adds acid and churns and stores food

Gallbladder stores bile

Small intestine absorbs nutrients

Colon—water is absorbed here

Anus—feces are expelled through the anus

Rectum—feces are formed here

defecation (a bowel movement), the waste is moved into the rectum and is then eliminated through the anus.

Daily fluid intake and loss

The intestines are capable of both absorbing and secreting fluids. Overall, it is estimated that nine liters (around nine quarts) of fluid pass through the intestines each day, of which only around two liters (two quarts) are derived from food and drink. The other seven liters (seven quarts) are secreted by the body itself, in the form of saliva, bile, and the juices of the stomach, pancreas, and intestine.

These secretions provide the necessary conditions for rapid digestion of nutrients and for optimal absorption of nutrients and minerals. Of the nine liters (nine quarts), approximately 8.8 liters or more are reabsorbed back into the blood, so that less than 200 grams (7 fluid ounces) of water are excreted in the stools each day.

The intestines are therefore efficient, reabsorbing as much as 98 percent or more of the water and minerals that pass through them. If anything prevents this from happening, so that less than 98 percent of water is reabsorbed, then stool output will be more watery and you will have diarrhea.

The large intestine

Normally, in the colon, the liquid material entering from the small intestine becomes solid as water is absorbed from it. This solid is then stored until it is convenient for you to move your bowels.

If you are an adult consuming a typical western diet, about 90 percent of the 1.5 liters (1 1/2 quarts) or so of

The digestive process and daily fluid intake and loss

Liquid is added as digestive juices in the mouth, stomach and duodenum. The intestines both absorb and secrete fluid. Overall, it is estimated that nine liters of fluid pass through the intestines each day. Only around two liters of this comes from food and drink. The other seven liters are secreted by the body itself, in the form of saliva, bile, and juices of the stomach, pancreas, and intestine. The intestines are very efficient, reabsorbing as much as 98 percent or more of the water and minerals that pass through them.

Key to diagram on opposite page

——— Oral intake
——— Saliva
——— Bile secretion
——— Gastric juices
——— Pancreatic secretions
——— Intestinal secretions
——— Reabsorption of water in intestines

The daily intake of water and the secretions within the body are efficiently absorbed by the gastrointestinal tract.

Source	Quantity of water
Oral intake	2,000 ml
Salivary glands	1,500 ml
Stomach	2,500 ml
Bile	500 ml
Pancreas	1,500 ml
Intestine	1,000 ml
Total water presented to the intestines	9,000 ml
Expelled in feces	200 ml
Absorbed by the intestines	8,800 milliliters (ml)

The digestive process and daily fluid intake and loss (contd)

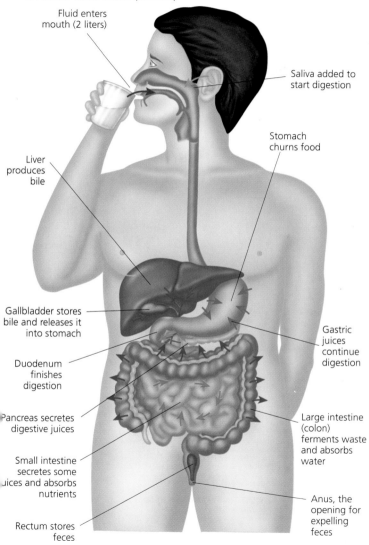

Fluid enters mouth (2 liters)

Saliva added to start digestion

Stomach churns food

Liver produces bile

Gallbladder stores bile and releases it into stomach

Gastric juices continue digestion

Duodenum finishes digestion

Pancreas secretes digestive juices

Large intestine (colon) ferments waste and absorbs water

Small intestine secretes some juices and absorbs nutrients

Anus, the opening for expelling feces

Rectum stores feces

The role of the intestines

Partially digested material enters the small intestine from the stomach. Liquid material enters the colon (large intestine) from the small intestine. It progressively solidifies as water is absorbed from it.

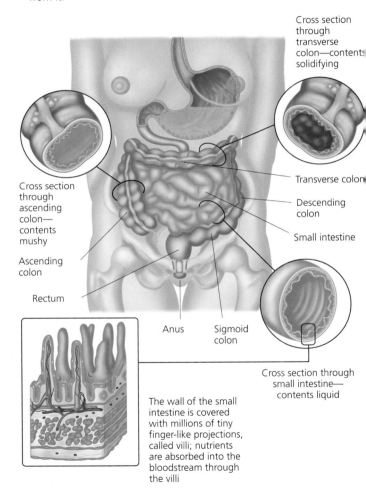

Cross section through transverse colon—contents solidifying

Transverse colon

Descending colon

Small intestine

Cross section through ascending colon—contents mushy

Ascending colon

Rectum

Anus

Sigmoid colon

Cross section through small intestine—contents liquid

The wall of the small intestine is covered with millions of tiny finger-like projections, called villi; nutrients are absorbed into the bloodstream through the villi liquid reaching your colon in a 24-hour period are absorbed. This leaves 200 milliliters (7 ounces) of semi-solid material to be excreted.

Food spends around 1 to 3 hours in the stomach, 2 to 6 hours in the small intestine, and 12 to 48 hours in the colon. Normally, it passes through the colon relatively slowly so as to allow fluid to be absorbed. The time it takes for food to pass through the entire system will vary from person to person and with diet.

Powerful muscle contractions propel solidified stool into the lower (sigmoid) colon and rectum several times a day. Defecation ultimately occurs as a result of complex interactions between sensory and motor nerves within the gut wall and the central nervous system. This interaction stimulates the muscles which empty the rectum. The muscles in the pelvis and rectum contract and the ring of muscle that controls the anus (the anal sphincter) relaxes in a coordinated way. Transit times through the colon are usually shorter in men than in women, and men's stools are heavier.

Progress of food through the body

After swallowing, food is moved by muscular contractions through the digestive system. The time spent in each part depends on the stage of digestion. It also varies with food type and quantity, and from day to day. The usual total time can vary from 15 hours to 5 days.

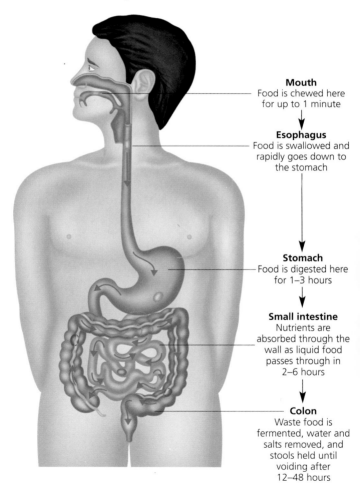

Mouth
Food is chewed here for up to 1 minute

Esophagus
Food is swallowed and rapidly goes down to the stomach

Stomach
Food is digested here for 1–3 hours

Small intestine
Nutrients are absorbed through the wall as liquid food passes through in 2–6 hours

Colon
Waste food is fermented, water and salts removed, and stools held until voiding after 12–48 hours

KEY POINTS

■ The gastrointestinal tract extends from the mouth to the anus; it digests and absorbs food and liquids and propels them along by muscle contraction

■ The small and large intestines are very efficient at absorbing fluid, so that most people excrete no more than 200 milliliters (7 ounces) of stool per day; if absorption is impaired, the result is diarrhea

■ The large intestine consists of the colon, rectum, and anus; transit through the colon is slow, which helps absorption of fluid

■ Muscle contractions move solid stool into the lower colon and rectum several times a day

■ Defecation occurs as a result of the interaction of several different parts of the nervous system, which cause the pelvic and rectal muscles to contract and the anal sphincter muscles to relax

What are the symptoms?

How do doctors diagnose IBS?

As there is no laboratory or other test that confirms the diagnosis of IBS, doctors have to rely on the symptoms alone. These vary from person to person, but there are three main types.

The predominant symptom may be abdominal pain with constipation, or the main problem may be abdominal pain with diarrhea. Also, both types of bowel disturbances can occur in an alternating pattern accompanied by abdominal pain.

Additional symptoms may include abdominal bloating and/or distension, gas, and unpredictable, erratic bowel actions varying from day to day.

There are some sex differences: straining and passage of hard stools may occur more commonly in women. In contrast, men are more likely to have frequent, loose stools.

As IBS can be diagnosed only from a collection of symptoms, doctors use certain criteria to help them.

Symptoms of IBS

The symptoms vary from person to person.

There are three main types:

1. Constipation predominant
2. Diarrhea predominant
3. Constipation and diarrhea together, accompanied by abdominal pain

Additional symptoms may include:

- Bloating and/or abdominal distension
- Unpredictable, erratic bowel actions varying from day to day

The Rome criteria

An international team of gastroenterologists has developed a set of symptoms to help define IBS, known as the Rome criteria. These recommend that a diagnosis of IBS be made when someone has experienced at least 3 months, with onset at least 6 months previously, of recurrent abdominal pain or discomfort associated with two or more of the following features:

1. The pain is relieved with defecation.
2. Onset of pain is associated with a change in frequency of passing stools.
3. Onset of pain is associated with a change in form (appearance) of stools.

While not all people with IBS fit these criteria, the majority do. Some people with other gastrointestinal disorders may also meet the Rome criteria but will have other symptoms not seen in IBS (such as fever or bloody stools) that allow doctors to tell the difference. People with constipation as the main symptom may have fewer than three bowel movements a week, with hard or lumpy stools. In contrast, those with diarrhea as the main symptom may have three or more bowel movements in a day with loose (mushy) or watery stools. A large percentage of patients also have alternating bowel habits, with hard and loose stools of variable frequency. The diagnosis of IBS is strengthened by the occurrence of further symptoms as listed below.

Other symptoms seen in IBS

Other symptoms include:

- straining during bowel movements
- urgency (having to rush to have a bowel movement)
- having a feeling of incomplete bowel movement
- passing mucus or slime with the bowel movement
- having abdominal fullness, bloating or swelling.

Other gastrointestinal features

The majority of people with IBS also have indigestion (also called dyspepsia). This consists of eating-related upper abdominal pain that doesn't change with bowel movements. Symptoms can vary over the years from being mainly bowel-type to mainly indigestion-type symptoms.

Non-gastrointestinal features

A wide range of non-gastrointestinal features, including bladder, muscle, or mood symptoms, may also be associated with IBS (see box on page 18).

Quality of life

Medically speaking, IBS is not a life-threatening condition. However, if you are a sufferer you will know how heavily it can restrict your social activities and reduce your quality of life. Chronic food-related pain may mean that you have to avoid eating out with friends or family. Fears about the need to move your bowels frequently or having bowel incontinence (leakage of stool) may seriously limit what you feel able to do.

Restricting activities

Over 40 percent of people with IBS say that they avoid some activities as a result of their symptoms. Examples are: traveling, socializing, sexual intercourse, domestic and leisure activities, or eating certain foods. Often it is this disruption to normal life rather than individual symptoms as such that determines how a person rates the severity of their condition.

Effects on well-being

People with IBS often also experience anxiety and disturbed sleep, with associated lethargy and an inability to get on with their lives. These symptoms can easily start to dominate a sufferer's existence.

Being unsure of the cause of the symptoms can add to the stress. If your doctor is unable to diagnose the cause of your symptoms easily, you are likely to be worried.

Non-gastrointestinal features of IBS

A wide range of other problems may occur along with the more typical ones of IBS. Women may have gynecological problems; there may be a problem passing urine or other symptoms that affect well-being.

Gynecological symptoms

- Painful periods (dysmenorrhea)
- Pain after sexual intercourse (dyspareunia)
- Premenstrual tension

Urinary symptoms

- Frequency—needing to urinate often
- Urgency—not being able to wait to urinate
- Passing urine at night (nocturia)
- Incomplete emptying of bladder

Other symptoms

- Back pain
- Headaches
- Unpleasant taste in the mouth
- Poor quality of sleep
- Constant tiredness
- Depression
- Anxiety
- Fibromyalgia

Not all doctors are familiar with the criteria for IBS and making the diagnosis can sometimes take several visits, or even an appointment with a specialist (a gastroenterologist). Sometimes, especially if you are a woman, you may end up having unnecessary surgery in an attempt to improve persistent and unexplained pain symptoms. This may be removal of the gallbladder or uterus. However, surgery could even make your existing disorder worse. It may also create its own specific postoperative complications, such as pain in the operation scar and adhesions (internal scarring causing cramping pains), so making the correct diagnosis before surgery is very important.

KEY POINTS

■ Your doctor will diagnose IBS if you meet the Rome criteria and do not have any other serious symptoms

■ A wide range of nongastrointestinal features is associated with IBS, for example, gynecological, urinary, musculoskeletal, and psychological symptoms

Understanding pain

What causes pain?

Having abdominal pain or discomfort is one of the key features of IBS. In spite of this, tests show that there is no structural abnormality of the intestines in IBS. So what causes the pain?

Pain is often a sign that you are doing something that may damage your body—for example, picking up a hot saucepan handle—or it may remind you that you already have damage from a burn or a bruise, and that your body needs time to heal. While IBS causes no damage to the body, the pain still occurs. Throughout the body, there are sensitive nerves which, when stimulated or irritated, send messages to the brain that are perceived as pain. Pain is primarily a protective mechanism, alerting you to the fact that something is wrong. It is often this that makes you consult a family doctor or general internist—and once the cause is dealt with it has served its purpose.

Pain is described as acute when it has started

recently (and often suddenly) and chronic if you have had it for a considerable length of time.

Types of abdominal pain

Doctors often find it difficult to distinguish between pain caused by a structural abnormality or disease (organic pain) and pain that does not appear to result from any identifiable structural changes or disease processes as in IBS (functional pain).

Functional pain

The term "functional pain" comes from the idea that the pain is the result of changes in the function of part of the body. Functional pain can be just as severe and disabling as organic pain—for example, women may describe their attacks of functional pain related to IBS as worse than that of childbirth.

Most people with IBS experience functional abdominal pain caused by disturbed bowel action. The term "functional abdominal pain" covers pain originating from any site within the abdominal cavity, including the gastrointestinal tract. Women seem to experience it more than men, particularly around the time of their periods, when hormonal changes affect muscle activity in the intestines.

Is the pain organic or functional?

Even an experienced doctor may sometimes find it difficult to tell whether your pain is organic or functional. Nevertheless, it is important that the distinction is made, to avoid any possibility of an organic disease (such as a bowel tumor) being wrongly diagnosed as a functional disorder (for example, as IBS).

The problem for the doctor is to distinguish the two types of pain without subjecting you to a series of tests that may be intensive, often uncomfortable, occasionally dangerous, and usually expensive. Such tests are not needed for someone with nonorganic, functional pain.

On the other hand, doctors have to take care not to dismiss too quickly someone who may have organic pain. Throughout the rest of the book, I shall explain how doctors use guidelines to help them choose the right approach.

What triggers abdominal pain?

Abdominal organs are usually insensitive to many stimuli that would be very painful if applied to the skin. Cutting, tearing, or crushing of the gut, for example, does not result in pain.

However, the nerve endings of pain fibers in the muscular walls of the gut are sensitive to stretching or tension. This means that excessive distension or tight contractions (spasm) in the gut wall will trigger pain.

Types of pain in IBS

There are many different terms to describe pain. Those most often used in IBS are described below.

- Acute: short-term, brief
- Chronic: long-term
- Functional: caused by abnormal functioning
- Visceral: felt in the abdomen
- Referred: felt somewhere other than the source

Visceral and referred pain

There are two types of abdominal pain that can occur in IBS. One is visceral pain (pain from the internal organs of the abdomen and intestines). The other is referred pain, which is felt in a different part of the body to the part that triggers the pain.

Visceral pain

Visceral pain is felt in the abdomen as a result of some form of stimulus within the gut itself. The pain is usually dull and is focused mostly somewhere along a line down the middle of the abdomen. It may be higher up or lower down, depending on where the nerve supply to the affected organ originates.

When healthy volunteers took part in experiments in which a balloon was inflated in different parts of the gut, the pain was felt in the midline of the abdomen. In addition:

- Pain arising from distension of the esophagus was perceived behind the breastbone.

- Pain from stimulation of the first part of the small intestine (called the duodenum) was felt between the lower ribs in the midline of the abdomen.

- Pain from the lower part of the small intestine (called the jejunum and ileum) was felt around the navel.

- Pain resulting from distension of the colon was felt in the midline of the lower abdomen.

In these studies there was no mention of pain caused by the balloons being felt anywhere outside the abdominal area. The location of pain felt by people with functional abdominal pain, however, is

Common myths about chronic pain

If they can't find a reason for my pain it must all be in my head!

Sometimes the cause of pain isn't clear—but the pain is still very real. Fortunately there is a lot that you can do to help yourself live with pain, even if you do not know the cause.

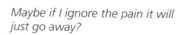

Maybe if I ignore the pain it will just go away?

No! Some effort and learning are necessary to manage pain effectively.

Perhaps I am suffering with this pain because I am a bad person?

Long-lasting (chronic) pain isn't a punishment for your past. But the things that you do and the way that you behave have an important effect on your self-esteem and the way that you feel.

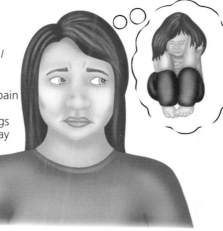

Common myths about chronic pain (contd)

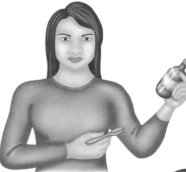

There are drugs that can cure pain.

Drugs can be effective in relieving pain. No drugs cure pain permanently.

Some people pretend to have pain as an excuse not to work or to get sympathy.

A few people may fake pain, but most sufferers of chronic pain only want relief.

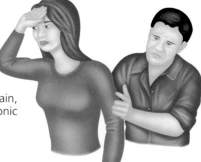

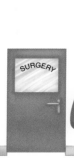
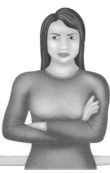

My doctors don't care, otherwise they would do something about my pain.

Your doctors will do everything that they can to assist you and relieve your pain. If they aren't completely successful, it isn't because they don't care.

much less clear-cut and often occurs outside the abdomen.

Referred pain

Referred pain is felt in an area that may be some distance away from the area where it is actually being caused. The nerves that sense pain from two regions of the body may be sent to your brain along the same pathway, sometimes causing the brain to interpret the source of the pain incorrectly. One example is pain caused by gallstones which is often felt between the shoulder blades even though the gallbladder is in the left side of the upper abdomen.

IBS patients may have referred pain in the back, chest, or legs. Referred pain may be felt in the skin or deeper tissues, but is usually confined to one particular area. Sometimes, the skin covering the painful region becomes unusually sensitive, and underlying muscles may feel tender or painful.

Pain threshold

The pain threshold is the level of tolerance at which someone perceives discomfort as pain. Some people have a low pain threshold and can tolerate less discomfort than others with a high pain threshold.

Your pain threshold is a subjective factor which can vary from time to time. It depends on the circumstances, your mood, the cause of the pain, and many other influences.

What can influence the severity of IBS symptoms?

Various factors can play a part in determining the severity of the symptoms of IBS; some relate to the illness itself, others to individual circumstances.

These include:

Psychological factors
Worry about your illness
Impaired ability to express emotions
Stress levels
Depression, anxiety, or panic attacks

The form your condition takes
Chronic (long-lasting) or intermittent
Unusual symptoms
Symptoms poorly controlled

Your circumstances
Poor social circumstances
Attitudes of relatives and friends
Sexual abuse as a child
Work and personal satisfaction
Economic gains from having an illness
Medical investigation and treatment

KEY POINTS

- Pain is a sensation felt when nerve impulses from the body are transmitted to the brain

- Pain may be acute (sudden onset) or chronic (long-term)

- Pain may be organic or functional; people with IBS have functional abdominal pain

- Pain may be felt in the abdomen (visceral) or somewhere unrelated (referred)

- Your pain threshold is influenced by your circumstances, mood, the cause of your pain, and many other factors

Causes of IBS

What triggers IBS?

The gastrointestinal tract is designed to digest food and propel the unabsorbed waste products to the end of the intestines for excretion. It does this by coordinated contraction and relaxation of the muscles in the bowel wall.

Although we do not completely understand the cause of IBS, one factor is disordered contractions of these bowel muscles. It is because the abnormalities involve bowel function, rather than any structural damage or abnormality, that IBS is often described as a functional disorder.

Why do some people develop IBS, whereas others do not? We do not know all the answers to that question, although some factors have been identified that are associated with an increased likelihood that an individual will have IBS. The main factors are:

- psychological factors
- abnormal activity of the bowel muscles and nerves
- increased sensitivity of the gut

- gastrointestinal infections
- diet, food intolerance

Who consults a doctor?

By no means everyone with symptoms consistent with IBS consults their doctor; the proportion ranges from 10 to 50 percent, and is influenced by age and sex. Some people find that their symptoms are troublesome whereas others pay them little attention.

Studies that have looked at the reasons why people consult their doctor have found both physical and psychological differences between those who seek medical care and those who do not. As you might expect, people with more symptoms and more severe pain are more likely to see a doctor, as are those with psychological symptoms such as anxiety and depression.

Psychological factors

People with IBS symptoms who do not consult a doctor are no more or less likely to experience psychological symptoms than those who don't have the condition. Around 8 to 15 percent of people who consult their doctor about their IBS symptoms have psychological symptoms, which is only a slightly higher percentage than among people without IBS.

Psychological symptoms are much more common, however, in people who are referred to a gastroenterologist. They also seem to be more common in people with IBS who are hospitalized than in a comparable group of people with an inflammatory bowel disease (IBD) such as Crohn's disease or ulcerative colitis.

How the bowel muscles work

When the muscles in the bowel wall contract, they move the contents along. When short sections contract and then relax, the contents move back and forth. If the contractions follow each other in a wave along the length of the bowel, the contents are moved towards the rectum. The difference is not in the strength of the contraction but in whether it keeps moving in the same direction, towards the rectum.

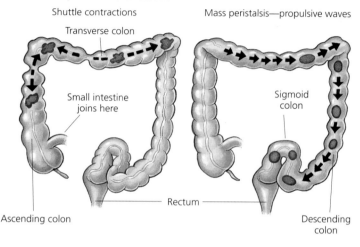

Shuttle contractions

Mass peristalsis—propulsive waves

Transverse colon

Small intestine joins here

Sigmoid colon

Ascending colon

Rectum

Descending colon

Several studies have also found a link between the onset of IBS symptoms and a preceding stressful event such as employment difficulties, bereavement, marital stress, or an operation for a different condition. Some studies have also found links between the development of IBS symptoms and social problems relating to work, finances, housing, or personal relationships.

These findings suggest that an individual's mood and emotions influence the way they respond to their symptoms (for example, whether they consult a doctor), as well as having a direct effect on their intestines. Stress has also been shown to play an important role in causing intestinal pain. Nevertheless, despite these findings, many people with IBS do not have any obvious psychological symptoms.

Depression and IBS

Around 10 to 15 percent of people with IBS who are referred to gastroenterology clinics are found to have a serious depressive illness and a minority of these may even be suicidal. This is why your doctor will want to ask you about symptoms that might suggest that you are depressed—such as sleep disturbance, unhappy mood, and changes in energy levels. However, the detection of depression is sometimes more difficult and, if your doctor is concerned, you may be referred for a full psychiatric assessment. If depression is present, recognized, and treated, IBS symptoms may improve or even resolve, even if severe.

Influence of mood on the gut

When you're depressed, the passage of waste matter throughout your whole gut is likely to be delayed. In contrast, anxiety is associated with accelerated passage of the digestive contents through the small bowel.

Most people have, at some time or other, experienced cramps and diarrhea caused by major anxiety. Acute stress also accelerates the passage of bowel contents through the small intestine and speeds up the working of the whole colon, so you have to move your bowels more often, whether or not you have IBS.

Research has shown that pain may be made less distressing by techniques such as relaxation and hypnosis. On the other hand, hyperventilation (rapid breathing that occurs during anxiety and panic attacks) has been shown to lower your pain threshold, so that any pain becomes more troublesome.

Abnormal activity of the bowel muscles and nerves

The workings of your bowels are controlled by several different parts of your nervous system. Changes in the activity of the nerves that supply the gut have been found in people with IBS. Psychological factors can affect these nerves and so can alter the speed at which intestinal contents pass through the bowels.

People who are constipated, including those with IBS for whom this symptom predominates, seem to have weaker and fewer contraction waves in their colonic muscle. Studies have generally shown fast passage of bowel contents in diarrhea-predominant IBS and slow transit time in constipation-predominant IBS. Some people with IBS may also experience abnormalities in small bowel contraction.

Abnormal bursts of nerve and muscle activity in the colon have been linked to episodes of pain in some individuals. In people with functional abdominal pain, the normal stresses of everyday life may provoke unusual muscle and nerve reactions in the stomach and small intestine.

Despite these observations, the relationship between nerve–muscle disturbances in the gut and abdominal pain is not clear-cut. Nor is it known whether such disturbances are the result of an abnormality in gut muscle or nerve activity or whether they are triggered by signals from the brain.

Gastrocolonic response

When we eat, our food stimulates an increase in colonic nerve and muscle activity, which is called the gastrocolonic response or reflex. This effect is one of the main reasons why a baby tends to fill his or her diaper just after a meal. This reflex is mainly stimulated by the fat content of food which explains why people with IBS can experience pain or urgency to go to the

The gastrocolonic response

When we eat, our food stimulates an increase in colonic nerve and muscle activity, called the gastrocolonic response. This effect is one of the main reasons why babies tend to fill their diapers after a meal.

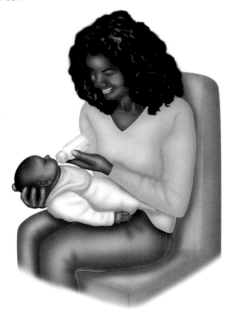

bathroom after eating, especially after eating fatty foods.

Increased sensitivity of the gut

Studies have been made using balloons inflated in parts of patients' guts to study the pain responses of people with IBS. These have shown that IBS patients are more sensitive than others to distension (or stretching) of the bowel.

In people with IBS, this abnormal sensitivity has been found in all parts of the gastrointestinal tract (esophagus and small and large intestines). It was also found that trigger areas for the production of pain may occur in the upper, mid, and lower gut in the same person.

Pain may be experienced anywhere in the abdomen. It may also be referred to various parts of the body away from the abdomen, such as the back, thighs, and arms.

People with functional abdominal pain resulting from IBS have increased sensitivity to the pain caused by the gut being distended with gas, yet their reactions to pain stimuli in other parts of the body are unaffected. They may describe gut stimuli as unpleasant or painful at lower levels of intensity than people who do not have IBS. No one knows why this should be the case, but the explanation probably originates in the brain and the way that different types of painful stimuli are perceived.

Gastrointestinal infections

Sometimes, symptoms of IBS can start after an acute episode of vomiting and diarrhea. Persistent problems with bowel function affect around one in four people after food-poisoning caused by bacteria such as Campylobacter, Shigella, and Salmonella species.

Factors that make persisting symptoms more likely include:

- female sex
- diarrhea lasting more than seven days
- vomiting leading to weight loss
- severe abdominal pain and mucus in the stools.
- higher anxiety levels
- higher number of stressful events in the six months before the illness.

These types of infection are responsible for long-term symptoms in up to 25 percent of people with IBS. Such people have a good outlook (prognosis), in that their symptoms often improve or disappear within a year or so.

Diet, food intolerance, and food allergy

Eating, especially eating fatty foods, triggers functional abdominal pain in around three of four people with IBS. It is important to distinguish this generalized intolerance to food from intolerance to specific foods, which may produce symptoms in certain individuals.

The role of true (specific) intolerance as a cause of IBS is debatable. True food intolerance is an adverse reaction in the intestines to a particular food and will occur every time a person eats that particular food. One example of this is excess gas and diarrhea as a result of lactose intolerance (inability to digest the sugar in milk, see page 38).

Food allergy, by contrast, brings on immediate symptoms whenever the individual eats the trigger food, such as strawberries or oysters. These allergic symptoms may involve the digestive system (such as vomiting), but they often affect other parts of the body, causing a rash, an attack of asthma, or a running nose.

Food intolerance

Studies were made that tested people's response to individual foods by excluding them from the people's diets and then reintroducing them one at a time. These studies found specific food intolerance in between a third and two-thirds of people with IBS. Patients with IBS appear to be more likely than those without IBS to have bowel symptoms in reaction to specific foods. Based on questionnaires sent to a large group of people in Minnesota, foods that seem to be most bothersome include dairy, beans, chocolate, nuts, and spicy foods.

Some people develop typical IBS symptoms such as bloating, cramps, and diarrhea after eating carbohydrates that they are unable to absorb. Examples are lactose (milk sugar) and fructose (fruit sugar). If they are not absorbed, they may ferment in the gut and produce gas. Excluding these from the diet can reduce symptoms and also reduce colonic gas production.

Reduced production of lactase—an enzyme that breaks down lactose—in the lining of the small intestine can develop in adults and is very common. It is estimated to affect 10 percent of those of northern European descent, rising to 75 percent in African-Americans, and 90 percent of people of Chinese descent.

People taking a substantial amount of lactose (equivalent to more than one cup (250 ml/9 fl oz) of milk per day) can expect to benefit if they reduce their consumption. On the other hand, those with lower lactose intakes may not, because a low intake does not usually cause symptoms of intolerance.

Elimination diets

Elimination diets (that is, diets that exclude all but a single type of fruit, a single type of meat, a single vegetable, and so on) improve symptoms in up to two-thirds of people with IBS but are very difficult to follow and require careful monitoring by a dietician to assure good nutrition.

More practical elimination diets, which impose less drastic restrictions on what you can eat, have been developed. These exclude only foods that are commonly implicated in food intolerance. These diets have a lower success rate but are easier to follow.

Whether diets for food intolerance are really worthwhile is hard to assess. This is because of the placebo response (in which you feel better just because you are expecting to). When given nothing but blended foods through a tube passing from the nose into the stomach, only 6 of 25 people with IBS correctly recognized that they had been given one of the foods that seemed to trigger their intolerance. Other influences, such as the social, psychological, and physical aspects of eating, are likely to play an important role. People often develop fears or anxiety about certain foods from past experiences that may effect how they respond to trying the food again. These other factors are likely to be at least as significant as the direct effects of individual foods on the gut.

Specific food intolerance appears to be the cause of symptoms in a small number of people with IBS. If your doctor suspects that this may be so in your case, you should preferably be referred to a specialist center for evaluation by a gastroenterologist, nutritionist, and possibly an allergist.

Food allergy

True food allergy is much less common than food intolerance and is usually not difficult to recognize. This is especially so when eating a particular food (or foods) is associated with a rash, asthma, a running nose, or more severe symptoms.

Such allergies often give a high incidence (70 percent) of positive results to allergy tests such as skin-prick and blood tests. Skin-prick tests are more likely to be positive if your symptoms start immediately after eating the suspect food than if they develop only some hours later. If you have this type of allergy, you are more likely to see a specialist in immunology rather than a gastroenterologist because your doctor is unlikely to think that you have IBS.

Women and IBS

Most studies show that IBS is more common in women, and women also are more likely to seek the help of a doctor than men. Anxiety, depression, and stress are known to occur more often in women, and this may play a part in triggering symptoms. It is also possible that hormonal differences may contribute to the differences between the sexes. During menstruation, for example, IBS symptoms of abdominal pain, diarrhea, and gas tend to get worse in about half of women.

Women with IBS are also more likely than men to show increased sensitivity of the gut and three times

Skin-prick test for allergy

A skin-prick test involves the tester placing drops of the suspect allergens on the skin. The skin is then pricked through each drop with a fine needle. An allergic reaction produces a red, itchy weal.

Test area
being pricked

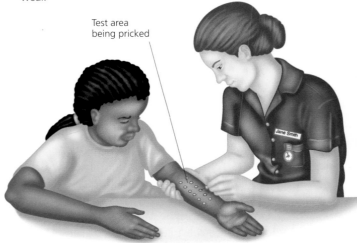

more likely than men to develop IBS after a gastrointestinal infection.

In 60 percent of women with IBS, pain may also sometimes be felt deep in the pelvis following intercourse. It can come on several hours after intercourse, particularly when the woman has constipation.

KEY POINTS

■ There are a number of factors, both physiological and psychological, that may make an individual more susceptible to IBS

■ Many people who develop IBS symptoms have had stressful experiences, such as work difficulties, bereavement, marital problems, gut infections, and operations, in the preceding months

■ People who develop IBS after a gut infection are more likely to have complete resolution of their symptoms

■ Three-quarters of people with IBS experience abdominal pain after eating, and a small proportion of them are intolerant to specific foods

■ Women are more prone to IBS than men

Getting a diagnosis

Consulting your doctor about abdominal pain or bowel symptoms

If you consult your doctor about abdominal pain or bowel symptoms, he or she will ask a variety of questions. These are designed to assess your symptoms, psychological state, and social circumstances, as well as your past family and personal history. Your doctor will give you a full physical examination. This may include a rectal examination and a test for blood in the stool. If you are under the age of 45 with typical symptoms of IBS (see page 15) and appear normal on physical examination, you may not need further investigations. Your doctor may suggest further tests to rule out other bowel problems (see pages 45–6) if you have weight loss, rectal bleeding, or symptoms responsible for night-time waking, or if your symptoms have come on suddenly over a relatively short period of time. If you have a family history of celiac disease (gluten intolerance) or iron deficiency anemia, your doctor may order blood tests to screen for celiac disease, which may produce symptoms similar to those of IBS. These examinations, together with what you have told the doctor about your symptoms, should be sufficient for a diagnosis to be made.

What happens if IBS is diagnosed?

If you have a typical history of IBS (your symptoms meet the Rome criteria, with or without negative test results), your doctor will usually confirm the diagnosis of IBS and give you a detailed explanation of the condition. He or she will reassure you that often symptoms improve on their own or at least become tolerable once you understand what is causing them.

Your doctor may also suggest simple lifestyle or dietary changes that may help (see pages 96–97). Depending on the type of symptoms that you have, your doctor may prescribe medications for the pain or bowel problems. You may also be recommended to use psychological therapies such as relaxation (see page 91).

If your symptoms continue, however, you should be seen regularly. It is important that a doctor makes the diagnosis of IBS—this is not a diagnosis you should ever make yourself.

When will your doctor refer you to a specialist?

This is likely to be necessary if you have developed bowel symptoms for the first time in later life, or if your symptoms are not typical of someone with IBS. If the initial recommendations for managing the symptoms aren't successful, or if you have had IBS for a while and your symptoms become worse, you may also be referred to a specialist, both to rule out other possible bowel conditions and to provide greater reassurance than your general internist can offer.

Further investigations

Upper endoscopy or colonoscopy (examining the upper or lower gut with a viewing instrument incorporating a tiny camera) may be recommended if the diagnosis of IBS is not clear. A sedative may be given before some types of endoscopy.

X-ray tests such as a CT (computerized axial tomography) scan, which can show detailed images of the internal organs, may be considered if there are unexplained findings on your physical exam or if you have unexplained weight loss.

Disadvantage of unnecessary investigations

Although extensive investigations may sometimes be necessary in difficult cases, most people don't really need them and they have a number of disadvantages. The tests may be inconvenient, uncomfortable, and expensive. The patient may also find the procedure demoralizing. Each test can increase your anxiety that there may be something seriously wrong and undermine your confidence in your doctor as each test produces negative results. It's not unusual for such investigations to detect another condition, such as a hiatus hernia (weakness in the diaphragm muscle) which may not, in fact, be responsible for your symptoms. Your doctor will usually be able to make a positive diagnosis based on your symptoms and a physical examination alone, without the need for extensive investigations.

Other symptoms

Although the diagnosis of IBS is based on the Rome criteria (see page 15), many people have additional symptoms, and you should mention these to you doctor, even if they seem unrelated. Common associated

Examination of rectum and colon with a colonoscope

The patient lies on the side with the knees bent, and usually has a mild sedative. The colon has previously been emptied by not eating, flushing out the contents using medication, and drinking large quantities of fluid. The flexible tube is inserted slowly along the colon and the small internal camera is connected to a video screen. In this diagram, the tube has reached the ascending colon.

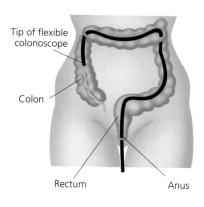

Tip of flexible colonoscope

Colon

Rectum

Anus

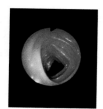

The display on the video screen shows the lining of the colon

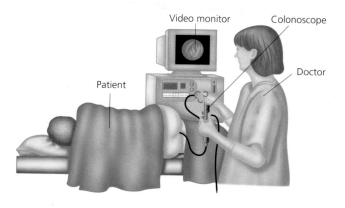

Video monitor

Colonoscope

Doctor

Patient

symptoms include nausea, vomiting, difficulty swallowing (dysphagia), and a feeling of fullness after eating.

You may notice the passage of undigested food in your stool. This is not usually significant; it usually consists of vegetable residues such as tomato or corn skins and merely indicates rapid transit through the gastrointestinal tract.

Non-gastrointestinal symptoms that people with IBS may also experience include frequent and urgent urination, and the feeling that you are unable to empty your bladder completely. Some people also experience back pain, an unpleasant taste in the mouth, a constant feeling of tiredness, and women may find intercourse painful. You should also discuss any problems you have been having with your mood, such as depression or anxiety, whether or not you think the symptoms may be causing, or caused by, your IBS.

Gynecological disorders

Your doctor will want to rule out other causes of lower abdominal and pelvic pain. For women, there are several gynecological disorders that may also cause pain in the lower abdomen. These disorders include:

- Pelvic inflammatory disease—inflammation of the tubes connecting the ovaries to the uterus (the fallopian tubes) and other structures in the pelvis.

- Endometriosis—in which cells from the lining of the womb are found in the pelvis.

- Pain that occurs in the middle of the menstrual cycle caused by swelling followed by rupture of a ripening egg follicle.

- Occasionally, pain in the lower abdomen and

disturbed bowel function could be a symptom of cancer of the cervix or the ovaries, and if your doctor thinks that either of these is a possibility, he or she may arrange for you to see a gynecologist. However, such cancers are very rare compared with IBS.

KEY POINTS

■ Your doctor will need as much information as you can give about your pain and other symptoms; it is worth making a note in advance so that you can tell him or her what triggers your symptoms, makes them worse or better, where the pain is, and whether it spreads to other parts of your body

■ Although some people may need further investigations in a gastroenterology clinic, often your general doctor will be able to make the diagnosis of IBS using the Rome criteria

■ When you see your general doctor, you will be asked questions about your lifestyle and any recent stressful events because psychological factors can play an important part in IBS

■ Most people with IBS can be treated after by their general doctor without needing to see a specialist

Constipation

What is a normal bowel habit?

People vary a lot in how often they move their bowels—usually between three times a day and three times a week. Interestingly, people living in different parts of the country and people from different ethnic backgrounds may have different bowel habits, possibly because of variations in their diets.

How the bowel works

The bowels work by a series of contractions and relaxations that mix the stool and propel it to the rectum, where it is stored untill you have a bowel movement. The activity of muscles in the colon can be changed by factors such as food and emotion.

When there are sufficient stools in the rectum to stretch it, this causes it to squeeze. At the same time, one of the muscles that keeps the anus closed (the internal sphincter muscle) relaxes. This all occurs without you being aware of it. Your brain then gets a signal that you need to have a bowel movement. When it is convenient to go, the stool is expelled when you

What does the bowel do?

Food passes from the stomach to the small intestine and then to the large intestine. We absorb nutrients from the digested food and most of the fluids that we have drunk. Some of this fluid is from intestinal secretions. The remaining waste matter (feces) is pushed to the rectum where we expel it through the anus. The bowel:

- Receives the food and liquids that we eat and drink
- Increases the amount of fluid in the intestines by liquid secretions from its lining
- Propels food contents from the stomach down its length to the anus
- Absorbs most of the nutrients from our food and drink into the bloodstream
- Excretes waste material as stools

push with the abdominal muscles, and relax the second muscle that keeps the anus closed (external sphincter muscle).

What is constipation?

Constipation has no universally accepted definition. A person can be considered to be constipated when fewer than three bowel movements happen in a week, if the stool is hard or lumpy, or if there is often a need to strain to pass a stool.

Constipation is hardly ever harmful in that you won't become "poisoned" or "dirty" if your bowels

What causes the usual types of constipation?

There are several simple explanations for most constipation. It is often caused by an unsuitable diet, bad bowel habits, or not using the muscles effectively:

- Diet: usually a lack of fiber (roughage) or water in the diet.

- Bad bowel habits: most people have an urge to use the bathroom once or twice a day. This often happens after a meal. If this urge is ignored, the stool dries out and becomes hard. The next bowel movement may then be difficult or painful.

- Uncoordinated straining: some people do not push effectively when trying to move their bowels and may fail to relax the muscles around the anus when they strain.

don't move regularly. Although constipation is not a disease, it is occasionally the symptom of an underlying disease. If you are constipated, your abdomen may feel uncomfortable or bloated and you may have a sense of fullness above your anus. Straining can lead to hemorrhoids (see page 57), which may bulge at the anus or bleed. Women may also find intercourse uncomfortable if the bowel is very full.

What causes constipation?

The most common causes of constipation are simple and are easily remedied. If your diet does not contain enough fiber, it is more difficult for your bowel to pass food along and keep the feces soft enough to pass easily.

Modern lifestyles make it difficult to respond immediately to the urge to empty the bowels. Ignoring this urge means that the feces are stored longer and they can become hard and dry.

Some people do not strain effectively or fail to relax the anal muscle to allow the rectum to empty. Retraining the use of the muscles will help this problem.

In a small number of people suffering from IBS, the colon moves much more slowly than usual, leading to very infrequent bowel movements.

What makes constipation worse?

Your bowel function is affected by many factors. These can make any tendency to constipation worse.

You must drink enough fluid each day—about two liters (two quarts or eight cups). If you become dehydrated, your feces will become harder.

Physical exercise massages the bowels and helps the passage along the gut, so inactivity will make any constipation worse.

What factors can aggravate constipation?

If you have a tendency to constipation, there are many factors that can make it worse:

- Dehydration: low fluid levels in the body
- Inactivity—lack of exercise
- Emotional upsets
- Painful anal conditions such as hemorrhoids
- Shift work
- Lack of bathroom facilities

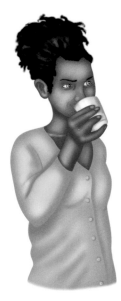

Drink plenty of fluids, at least four pints spread over the day.

Your emotions have a strong effect on your bowels. Anxiety can speed the passage along your bowels, but other emotions can slow it down and lead to constipation.

Painful conditions that affect the anus will aggravate any constipation. Hemorrhoids are swollen blood vessels around the anus which can be the result of straining to have a bowel movement, which you are more likely to do if you are constipated. When they are painful it makes it harder to move your bowels regularly.

Working hours can interfere with a regular bowel habit. You may have to be at work early in the morning and leave home before you have emptied your bowels.

Or you may work shifts that interfere with your normal body rhythm.

A lack of suitable bathroom facilities can aggravate constipation. Many people feel uncomfortable having a bowel movement at work or in public restrooms, so will ignore the urge to go until they are home.

What disorders cause constipation?

A number of organic and functional disorders can affect bowel movement. Any obstruction of the bowel as a result of scarring, inflammation, or the growth of a tumor can lead to constipation. The pressure of an enlarged uterus and other changes in pregnancy can affect bowel movement. An underactive thyroid gland often results in constipation. Any alteration in the nerves or muscles that control bowel movement, as happens in IBS, can lead to constipation.

What conditions and disorders may cause constipation?

There may be underlying organic or functional reasons for constipation:

- Obstruction to the bowels by scarring, inflammation, or a tumor
- Pregnancy
- Underactive thyroid gland
- Altered function in the nerves or muscles controlling bowel movement, such as in IBS

What medicines can cause constipation?

Some constipation can be a side effect of medication taken for another reason. This is usually explained on the patient information leaflet that comes with the medication:

- Antacids containing aluminum or calcium that are taken to fight indigestion
- Iron tablets (sometimes)
- Some pain-killers such as codeine
- Cough medicines that also contain codeine
- Some antidepressant drugs or sedatives
- Drugs that influence muscle function, such as some given for abdominal pain, bladder relaxation, or Parkinson's disease

What medicines cause constipation?

Medications all have some effects other than those for which we take them. One of the side effects is constipation. All side effects from medications should be explained on the patient information leaflet that comes with the medication. Those medications that are known to be likely to cause constipation are listed in the box above.

What is fiber and how does it help?

Fiber is found in the tough fibrous part of fruits and vegetables. In particular, it is found in the stalk and on the outside of fruits, seeds, or grains (bran is the outer covering of cereal grains, such as wheat, oats,

Hemorrhoids

Hemorrhoids are anal blood vessels that have been pushed down and may protrude from the anal canal. Hemorrhoids are caused by straining to pass a stool.

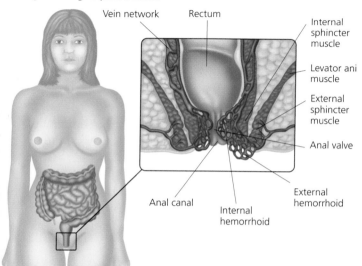

Vein network — Rectum — Internal sphincter muscle — Levator ani muscle — External sphincter muscle — Anal valve — External hemorrhoid — Anal canal — Internal hemorrhoid

and rye). It is also in the soft parts of fruits and vegetables that are not digested by the small intestine.

Much of the food that we eat is digested in the stomach and small intestine and is absorbed as nutrients. Fiber is not broken down in this way but passes to the large intestine (colon). Here it:

- acts like a sponge, soaking up water and keeping it in the stool

- provides material that encourages the multiplication of useful bacteria in the colon.

Both these effects make the stool larger, softer, and easier to pass. Bulky stools stimulate your gut wall, increasing the propulsive waves of contraction (peristalsis) so that they pass through more easily.

Dietary fiber is found only in foods that derive from plants—for example, cereals, fruits, and vegetables. It is not found in animal foods. So, if you need to increase your fiber intake, gradually start to use the foods listed on pages 58–61. If you already eat some of them, try to do so more often.

You may experience some increase in the amount of gas in the intestines (flatulence) and this may lead to abdominal discomfort at first. This should lessen as your body becomes used to the change in your diet. Drink plenty of fluids (at least 2 liters (2 quarts) per day) because the fiber will absorb water. It may be helpful to discuss what you eat with a dietitian.

Foods containing a good source of fiber

Many foods contain fiber. They are all foods derived from plants:

- Whole-grain bread: eat this regularly in preference to white bread. You could also try whole-grain muffins, biscuits, pita bread, and tortillas.

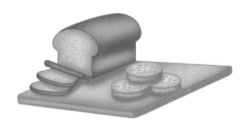

- Whole-grain and high-fiber breakfast cereals eaten on a daily basis. Look at the package labeling to determine which of the cereals you enjoy contain the highest amount of fiber.

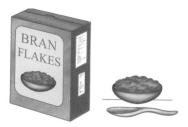

- Whole-wheat flour: try using equal quantities of whole-wheat flour and white flour in cooking (don't sift the flour).

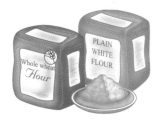

- Cookies and crackers: instead of cookies and crackers made with white flour, choose whole-wheat varieties.

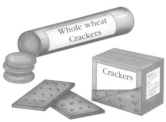

- Brown rice: this takes longer to cook than white rice but it is more nutritious.

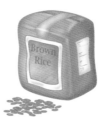

- Whole-wheat pasta: for example, spaghetti, macaroni, fettucini, lasagne.

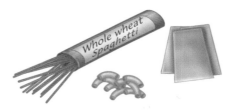

- Legumes: these include chickpeas (garbanzo beans), dried peas, beans, and lentils. Try using them in soups and to replace some of the meats in stews and casseroles. They can also be cooked, then eaten cold in salads.

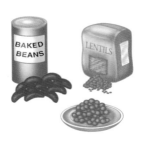

- Vegetables: especially brussels sprouts, spinach, and broccoli. Eat them lightly cooked and try crunchy side-salads with your main meal and lunchtime snack. Start with small amounts, as some people find these vegetables give them gas or cramping.

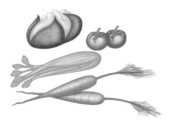

- Fruit: eat fresh, dried, or canned in natural juices. Prunes and prune juice are particularly good at relieving constipation. Add dried fruits to cereals and use them in baking.

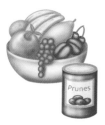

- Nuts and seeds: for example, sunflower seeds. Eat as a snack or use in salads or cooking.

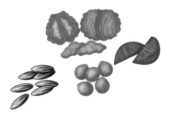

Dietary fiber, bran, and bulk-forming laxatives

Some people with IBS or functional abdominal pain benefit when their doctors prescribe a high-fiber diet, bran, or laxatives that add bulk to the stool (bulk-forming laxatives). Others, however, notice no change or even a deterioration in their symptoms.

Bran

Natural bran is the outer layer of the wheat grain. It adds fiber to the diet, but you should use it as a supplement only if your doctor or a dietitian advises you to do so. Start by adding one teaspoon to food or drink for three meals each day. Gradually increase the amount over the next few days if needed. One tablespoon of bran three times daily is usually enough to treat constipation. It may cause some flatulence when you first start to use it.

Bran can improve constipation significantly, but it can exacerbate diarrhea, abdominal pain, and urgency, so is not for all people with IBS.

Bulk-forming laxatives

Treatment intended to add bulk to the stools is likely to be effective for people who frequently pass small, hard stools or who pass only a painful, irregular stool every few days. A high-fiber diet alone is often ineffective and a bulking agent (a fiber source that swells in the bowels to provide bulk, such as ispaghula husk (psyllium) and methylcellulose) is usually required. Symptoms of gas and pain are sometimes aggravated by a sudden increase in dietary fiber, so this treatment isn't advisable for everyone. If your normal diet is low in fiber, try increasing your intake slowly and adjust the amount according to the way your system responds. Usually after a few weeks, the body gets used to the higher fiber content and the gas symptoms decrease. On the other hand, especially if your intake is very high and you are experiencing pain and distension, you may need to reduce your intake of fiber. Fiber must be taken with plenty of water if it is to be effective.

What if some foods don't suit me?

Some people with IBS find that legumes, nuts, dried fruits, and some vegetables cause a lot of gas or discomfort. If you find that these foods upset you, it may be better to avoid them.

Is it important to eat breakfast?

Yes. Eating breakfast helps your bowels to start working during the morning.

The best type of breakfast is a whole-grain or high-fiber cereal or some whole-grain toast. If you prefer a

Healthy eating can prevent weight increase

If you have to change what you eat to avoid constipation you may be worried about putting on weight. The foods that you will be recommended are not fattening in themselves. You just have to combine them in a healthy and balanced way.

General

- Use a low-fat spread
- Use a low-fat milk
- Exercise more

What should you weigh?

- The body mass index (BMI) is a useful measure of healthy weight
- Find out your height in inches (ins) and weight in pounds (lbs)
- Calculate your BMI like this:

$$BMI = \frac{\text{Your weight (lbs)}}{[\text{Your height (ins)} \times \text{Your height (ins)}]} \times 703$$

$$\text{e.g. } 23 = \frac{160 \text{ (lbs)}}{[70 \text{ ins} \times 70 \text{ ins}]} \times 703$$

- Males are recommended to try to maintain a BMI in the range 20.0 to 25.0
- Females are recommended to try to maintain a BMI in the range 18.7 to 23.8
- The chart below is an easier way of estimating your BMI. Read off your height and your weight. The point where the lines cross in the chart indicates your BMI

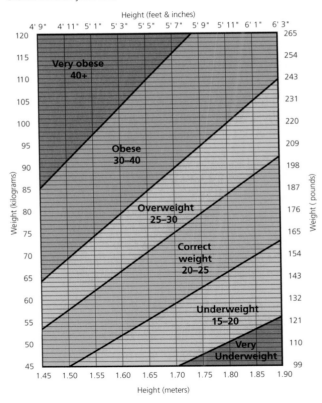

cooked breakfast, try oatmeal or another hot whole-grain cereal.

Will I put weight on if I eat more whole-grain bread, potatoes, and cereals?

Not if you cut down your intake of fat, fatty foods, sugar, and sweet foods, and eat in moderation. Small portions of bread, potatoes, rice, pasta, and cereals are not fattening in themselves, but they are if you serve them with fatty sauces or spreads

If you are worried about your weight, discuss this with your doctor and consider seeing a nutritionist. For more suggestions, look in your local library or bookstore for books about high-fiber, vegetarian, and whole-food cooking.

What if my bowels are not regular?

- Always try to go to the bathroom as soon as you feel the urge
- Try to do this as a routine, for example, as soon as you get up, or after breakfast
- Drink at least 2 liters (2 quarts) of fluid daily
- Eat more natural fiber
- Be as active as possible and exercise regularly
- Avoid laxatives unless recommended by your doctor
- Have your meals at the same time every day
- Ensure that you have access to good bathroom and restroom facilities

When should you see your doctor?

If constipation is not responding to these simple self-help measures and is causing you trouble, you should make an appointment to see your doctor. Any changes in bowel habit, either sudden or gradual, should also be reported to the doctor.

You should consult him or her quickly if there is bleeding when you move your bowels, or if you get new symptoms, such as abdominal pain or distension. You should also see your doctor right away if you suddenly become constipated for no apparent reason.

You will probably not need any tests, although your doctor may want to take a blood sample. This is to

Barium X-ray examination

Your doctor may arrange a barium X-ray examination of your bowel. Barium is a thick liquid that does not allow X-rays to pass through it, so it shows up well on X-ray pictures. It is given as an enema after a laxative has been taken to empty the bowel. X-ray pictures are then taken of the colon.

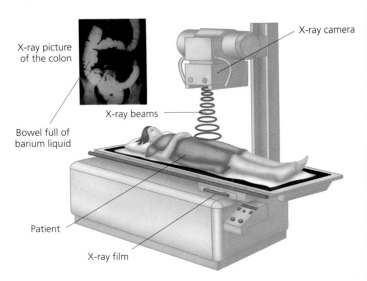

X-ray picture of the colon

Bowel full of barium liquid

X-ray beams

X-ray camera

Patient

X-ray film

make sure that you are not anemic and that your thyroid gland is working properly. If the constipation is very bad, your doctor may wish to check whether your colon is normal by arranging one of the following tests:

- A barium enema X-ray. This involves the insertion into the rectum of a harmless material which shows up on an X-ray, allowing the doctor to see any abnormalities.

- A sigmoidoscopy or colonoscopy (inserting a flexible viewing instrument so the doctor can see the interior of the colon)—see pages 44–7.

- Tests to check the function of the muscles around the anus.

Are laxatives useful?

Constipation is usually improved by a change in your diet, and drugs are therefore not needed. Occasional use of a suitable laxative is harmless, but some people become dependent on them. Laxatives can also cause abdominal pain and urgency. A few people will need to take laxatives regularly, but this should be done only on a doctor's advice.

The choice of laxatives includes the following:

- Stimulant laxatives: bisacodyl or senna which stimulate contraction of the bowel.

- Osmotic laxatives: mineral salts (magnesium citrate, magnesium hydroxide, polyethylene glycol). These retain water in the bowel, softening the stools and making them easier to pass.

- Lactulose or sorbitol sugars which humans cannot digest. They stay in the bowel and combine the properties of bulk and osmotic laxatives, though they can cause bloating side effects.

- Suppositories inserted into the rectum which soften the stool and stimulate bowel action.

- Enemas: a few people, especially those with severe nerve damage in the spine, have to use enemas in which a liquid solution is flushed into the lower bowel to wash it out.

With any laxative, it is important to keep up a good fluid intake—at least 2 liters (2 quarts) of fluid every day, more if possible.

Prescription medications

A few prescription medications are available for constipation and new ones are in development all of the time. If simple dietary measures, fiber, or occasional laxatives are ineffective, your doctor will discuss possible prescription medications for constipation.

Other treatments

Special tests may show that you have a problem coordinating straining to move the stools while relaxing the exit from the bowel (the anal sphincter). If you have this disorder, you may be helped by being trained in how to contract your abdominal muscles and relax those around your anus effectively.

This training can be supplemented by a device that enables you to tell whether your muscle is relaxed (biofeedback—see page 91), but most people don't need this. Training the muscles is, at present, limited to a few centers specializing in IBS or bowel motility.

If constipation is associated with emotional problems, counseling or similar treatment may help.

A small number of people require surgical treatment, but this is needed only by those with a definite abnormality of the large intestine.

KEY POINTS

■ Changing your diet and developing good bowel habits, together with increased exercise, will be enough for most people to relieve their constipation

■ Bulk-forming or osmotic laxatives are preferable to stimulant laxatives, which should be taken regularly only under medical supervision

■ If you are constipated, this does NOT mean that bodily wastes are being absorbed and damaging your health

■ If you are over 40 and for no obvious reason have sudden or gradual changes in bowel habit, you should see your doctor (especially if you have rectal bleeding or new abdominal symptoms such as distension)

Diarrhea

What is diarrhea?

Diarrhea means that there are frequent, loose, or liquid stools, sometimes accompanied by cramps and abdominal pain which lessens after a stool is passed:

- Acute diarrhea starts suddenly and lasts a short time.
- Chronic diarrhea affects the patient over a long period of time.

Some people pass frequent, small, solid stools with a sense of urgency. This is not true diarrhea and occurs when the rectum is irritable as in IBS or inflamed as in colitis.

What causes diarrhea?

You develop acute diarrhea when too much fluid is passed (secreted) from the bloodstream into the bowel, for example, in food poisoning or other types of bowel infections. Some laxatives work by provoking a similar response (osmotic laxatives).

Diarrhea may also be the result of your bowel

contents moving through your system too quickly so that less fluid is absorbed. This is one way in which anxiety produces diarrhea.

Drinking more liquid than your bowel can cope with can also cause loose stools. Although this seldom happens, it is one way in which drinking too much beer can cause diarrhea. Excessive amounts of alcohol can also have the same effect by irritating the bowel. Sometimes treatment with an antibiotic for an infection can result in acute diarrhea. You should make an appointment to see your doctor if acute diarrhea does not settle after a few days.

When diarrhea continues for months, the most likely cause is IBS, though a few less common disorders can cause similar symptoms. In the case of IBS, the bowel produces stools that are looser or more frequent than normal, but the bowel is not diseased. See your doctor promptly if you have severe diarrhea with dehydration (dry mouth, loose skin, sunken eyes) or if you are over the age of 60. You should ask for an early appointment with your doctor if liquid stools contain blood and/or if you are losing weight.

What will your doctor do?

After asking appropriate questions, and performing a general examination, your doctor will usually examine your rectum with a lubricated, gloved finger. Your doctor may:

- arrange a laboratory examination of stool samples to see if there is infection
- arrange blood tests
- arrange an examination of the interior of your colon using a flexible sigmoidoscope or colonoscope and

Examination of a stool sample

If your doctor asks for a stool sample to send to the laboratory you will be given a sample container. At the laboratory the sample will be examined under a microscope to look for any organisms that may cause infection.

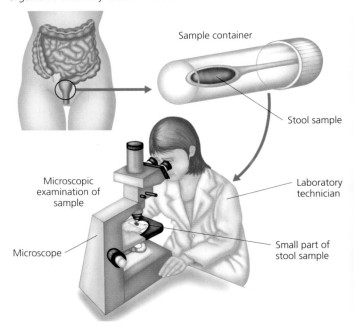

Sample container

Stool sample

Microscopic examination of sample

Laboratory technician

Microscope

Small part of stool sample

taking samples of the lining for examination if abnormalities are seen (see page 47).

Drug treatment

Anti-diarrheal drugs are helpful if you are passing stools very frequently. However, they may make abdominal discomfort worse and also your constipation worse if you have a tendency to alternate this with bouts of diarrhea. If taken at night, they may diminish the early morning stool frequency.

Taking a blood sample

A blood sample is usually taken by a nurse at your doctor's office or laboratory. A tourniquet around your upper arm makes the vein stand out. The nurse inserts a small needle into the vein and draws a small sample of blood up into the syringe.

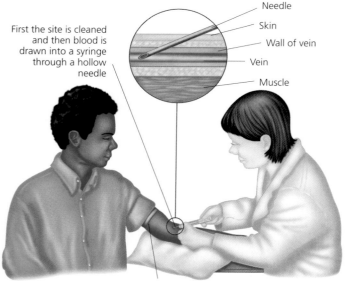

First the site is cleaned and then blood is drawn into a syringe through a hollow needle

Needle

Skin

Wall of vein

Vein

Muscle

A tourniquet may be applied to make the vein more prominent

The two common anti-diarrheal drugs—diphenoxylate (Lomotil, Lonox) and loperamide (Diasorb, Imodium)—are equally effective in most cases. You may find that one of them suits you better than the others or that one causes fewer side effects.

What is fecal incontinence?

Most of us take it for granted that we can control our bowels. We barely have to think about controlling the release of gas, or of liquid or solid stools from the bowel. We do not have "accidents," unless perhaps during a sudden severe bout of diarrhea.

Sometimes, however, control is lost because the bowel or the muscular ring (sphincter) around the exit from the anus does not function properly or the urgency to have a bowel movement is too strong. Bowel contents escape and this can be extremely embarrassing.

Fecal incontinence, also known as soiling, is the loss of stool, liquid or gas from the bowel at an undesirable time. It can occur at any age and may affect up to one in 20 people. It is certainly more common than was thought some years ago. Simple tests can usually show where the problem is, and treatment is often effective.

How do we normally control the bowel?

Normally the bowel and ring of muscle around the anus, the anal sphincter, work together to ensure that bowel contents are not passed until we are ready.

The sphincter has two main muscles that keep the anus closed. There is an inner ring (internal anal sphincter), which keeps the anus closed at rest, and an outer ring (external anal sphincter), which provides extra protection when we exert ourselves or when we cough or sneeze. These muscles, the nerves supplying them, and the sensation felt within the bowel and sphincter all contribute to the sphincter remaining tightly closed. This balance enables us to stay in control (or "continent").

What causes incontinence?

Fecal incontinence occurs most commonly because the anal sphincter is not functioning properly. Damage to the sphincter muscles or to the nerves controlling these

Controlling bowel opening

Feces are stored in the rectum with its muscular walls relaxed. The anal sphincter is contracted. When we are ready to empty our bowels, we contract the rectal muscles at the same time as relaxing the anal sphincter.

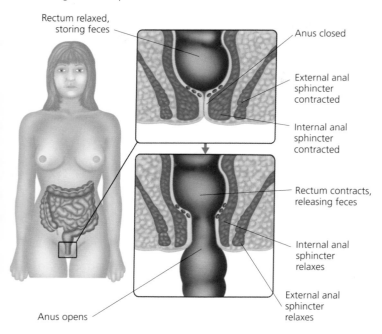

Rectum relaxed, storing feces

Anus closed

External anal sphincter contracted

Internal anal sphincter contracted

Rectum contracts, releasing feces

Internal anal sphincter relaxes

External anal sphincter relaxes

Anus opens

muscles, excessively strong bowel contractions, or alterations to bowel sensation can all lead to this disturbance of function.

Men and women of any age may be incontinent for various reasons:

- Children and teenagers—if they are born with an abnormal sphincter or if they have persistent constipation which can affect the sphincter through constant straining.

- Women, after childbirth—usually caused by a tear (hidden or obvious) in the sphincter muscles.

- People of any age who experience an injury or infection of the sphincter—they may be affected immediately or later in life.

- People who have inflammatory bowel disease or IBS—because the bowel is very sensitive and squeezes strongly.

- Elderly people—because of constipation and overflow from the bowel as a result of failing mental capacity, or of sphincter damage sustained when they were younger.

- People with disorders such as multiple sclerosis, stroke, and epilepsy—which result in damage to the nerves supplying the sphincter.

What tests may be needed?

Tests of sphincter function are relatively simple. They do not require preparation, and are quick to perform and usually pain-free. The strength of the muscles, sensation, and nerve function, for example, can all be tested using simple pressure-measuring devices.

An ultrasound scan can provide a clear picture of both the sphincter muscle rings, showing whether one or both are damaged. This test is not uncomfortable, takes only five minutes, and involves no radiation.

These tests are performed by doctors with a special interest in incontinence. If you need them you will be referred by your general doctor or gastroenterologist.

What is the treatment?

Anti-diarrheal drugs (see page 73) may be helpful when:

- the bowel is squeezing too strongly (an urgent need to get to the restroom quickly)
- the stool is very loose
- the sphincter muscles are weak.

These drugs can help in several ways:

- decrease movement in the bowel
- make the stool more formed
- make the sphincter muscle tighter.

When the sphincter has been injured, creating a gap in the sphincter muscles, an operation performed through the skin around the anus can often cure the problem. When there is nerve damage to sphincter muscles, a different operation to tighten the sphincter will sometimes help.

Techniques such as biofeedback (see page 91) are now available to retrain the bowel to be more sensitive to the presence of stool, so that the sphincter contracts when necessary.

KEY POINTS

■ Diarrhea means frequent, loose, or liquid stools; acute diarrhea usually settles by itself, whereas chronic diarrhea may be clearly due to IBS or may require further investigation

■ IBS is the most common cause of chronic diarrhea

■ Anti-diarrheal drugs, such as diphenoxylate (Lomotil, Lonox) and loperamide (Imodium, Diasorb), are usually effective

■ Fecal incontinence is quite common, especially in elderly people and in women who have had difficult and prolonged childbirth; simple tests can often identify these problems and various kinds of treatment are available

Related symptoms

Lump in the throat

Many people have felt a brief "lump in the throat," often with a dry mouth, usually during strong emotion, particularly grief—especially if they're trying not to cry. This is quite different from a condition called *globus hystericus*, which is the sensation of a lump in the throat associated with difficulty in swallowing. This sensation may be brought on by anxiety, especially if it leads to overbreathing (hyperventilation).

Difficulty in swallowing may also be a problem when acid comes up into the esophagus (known as "reflux"). This often affects people with IBS (see "Heartburn and related symptoms" on page 80). The difficulty in swallowing will usually disappear once the problem of reflux has been treated.

Nausea and vomiting

Nausea and vomiting can result from a wide variety of problems relating to the gut, nervous system, and hormone balance. If you also experience abdominal pain and have lost weight, your doctor will probably want to arrange tests to establish the underlying cause.

Nausea on its own, especially if you have been prone to it for some time or experience it repeatedly, is virtually never serious. If you have diabetes, it may be a sign that your stomach is emptying too slowly.

Your doctor may want to discuss possible psychological explanations because nausea and vomiting that occur shortly after a meal are often the result of excessive anxiety. This is especially likely if you have no other symptoms, such as weight loss, and if the results of an X-ray test, called an "upper gastrointestinal series," and endoscopy tests are normal.

Treatment involves identifying stress factors and helping you to try to deal with them better. Sometimes, you may be given drug treatment to relieve anxiety and to suppress the symptoms.

Heartburn and related symptoms

Around half of people with IBS have symptoms of heartburn. This is caused by the partially digested stomach contents flowing back up the esophagus (refluxing), which may result in an inflamed esophagus. Waterbrash, the regurgitation of a clear, very liquid saliva into the mouth, is unlikely to be caused by disease. If you have persistent heartburn, you may be referred to a gastroenterologist for an upper endoscopy (examination of the esophagus, stomach, and duodenum by inserting an instrument with a camera at its tip) to make sure there isn't another cause for your symptoms, such as a stomach ulcer.

If you have heartburn, this can usually be treated effectively by simple measures such as losing excess

The gastroscopy examination

A flexible tube is passed down the throat to examine the esophagus, stomach, and duodenum. The gastroscope can cause discomfort, so the patient is offered a throat spray or intravenous sedation. The gastroscope tube has a camera at its tip and the lining of the esophagus, stomach, and duodenum are viewed on a screen.

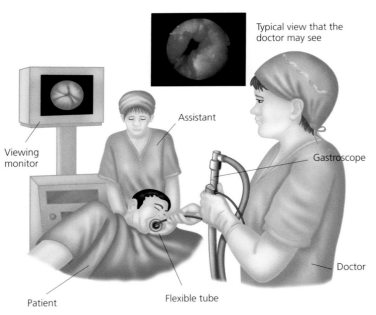

Typical view that the doctor may see

Assistant

Viewing monitor

Gastroscope

Doctor

Patient

Flexible tube

weight, taking an antacid or acid-blocking drug, and sleeping with the head of your bed raised a few inches (see page 83).

Feeling uncomfortably full, with discomfort around your upper abdomen, is not usually an indication that anything serious is wrong. However, you may be sent for an X-ray or upper endoscopy to be certain. "Butterflies" in your stomach and a "sinking feeling in

Gastro-esophageal reflux (heartburn)

Gastro-esophageal reflux (heartburn) occurs when the acidic stomach contents leak back into the esophagus, causing the symptoms that we know as heartburn.

Normal

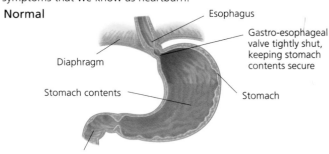

Esophagus

Gastro-esophageal valve tightly shut, keeping stomach contents secure

Diaphragm

Stomach contents

Stomach

Duodenum

Reflux

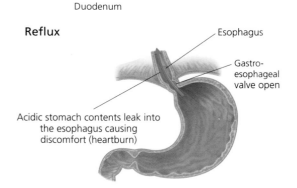

Esophagus

Gastro-esophageal valve open

Acidic stomach contents leak into the esophagus causing discomfort (heartburn)

After Medication

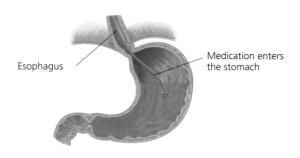

Esophagus

Medication enters the stomach

Avoiding heartburn at night

If you lie on a horizontal bed it is easier for your stomach contents to leak into the esophagus and cause heartburn. Sleeping on a bed raised slightly at the head end can avoid this.

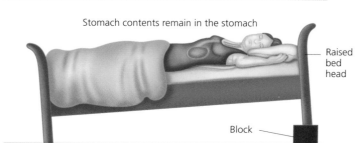

Stomach contents leak into the esophagus

Stomach contents remain in the stomach

Raised bed head

Block

the pit of the abdomen" are unpleasant but rarely symptoms of any serious disorder.

Gas

Many people are bothered by intestinal gas. It is useful to have a few facts about gas (see box on page 85).

Excess gas

One of the more interesting statistics about intestinal gas is that healthy people expel intestinal gas on average 14 times per day. In fact, it is probable that most people who think that they pass unusually large quantities are not that different in this respect from other people.

Although poor absorption and poor digestion may be responsible for gas production, organic disease is rarely a factor. Often those who are concerned about gas are particularly anxious and may have other emotional problems.

Factors such as timing, frequency, noise and smell, rather than total amount passed, may determine whether you perceive gas as a symptom. It can cause problems such as burping, belching, noisy intestinal rumblings, abdominal distension, pain, or passing embarrassing amounts of gas.

How would I know if I have excess gas?

There are two possible ways in which these symptoms can be caused. It may be an increase in the volume of gas in the gastrointestinal tract or it may be a reduction in the rate at which it is expelled or cleared.

An increase in the volume of intestinal gas may result from increased intake of swallowed air or enhanced production of gas in the colon by bacterial fermentation. A reduced rate of clearance of gas is most common in people who have long-term problems of excessive gas and bloating.

Some people form a normal amount of intestinal gas but the infusion of gas into their intestines produces more discomfort and pain than normal. This suggests that their symptoms are caused by an abnormal sensitivity of the gut rather than an abnormal stimulus.

Swallowing air

Everyone swallows some air along with saliva when they eat or drink. However, some of those who

Facts about gas

We often know little about intestinal gas—and even find it embarrassing. However, it is normal during digestion to produce gas.

Quantity of gas
Normal volume of gas in gastrointestinal tract = 150–200 ml (about 2/3 cup)

Normal total volume of gas passed per day = 1,000–1,500 ml (about 4–6 cups)

Major components of gas
Oxygen and nitrogen—from swallowed air

Hydrogen—from metabolism of carbohydrates

Methane—produced by bacteria in the gut

Smell of gas
The unpleasant smell of gas expelled through the rectum comes from bacterial fermentation of fiber in the colon. This depends on diet—some foods such as onions and garlic produce more "smelly" gas than others. The worst smells are of ammonia and sulfur-containing components.

complain of excess gas in the stomach take in two to three times as much air as fluid.

The habit of swallowing air even when not eating is known as aerophagia. Factors that may encourage it include mouth-breathing, ill-fitting dentures, canker sores, smoking, chewing gum, taking certain medications, eating too quickly, and emotional disturbance. Some people deliberately swallow air then belch, in an effort to relieve pain caused by esophageal reflux or other disorders. Your doctor will need to find out the reason why you are swallowing air in order to be able to treat the problem correctly. One trick that may prove useful in overcoming aerophagy and belching is to place a pen between your teeth. You can't suck air into your esophagus with a pen in your mouth!

Bacterial fermentation

Increased production of gas may result from excess bacterial fermentation of carbohydrates in your diet. In healthy people, this normally occurs in the colon. If you have a condition that impairs your digestion or that prevents you from absorbing food properly, it may also occur in the small intestine.

If you eat a high-fiber diet, especially one that includes a lot of fruits and vegetables, especially beans, this can result in fermentation. This, in turn, leads to an increased production of gas, particularly carbon dioxide and hydrogen.

Bacterial fermentation in the colon produces a number of smelly gases such as ammonia and hydrogen sulfide. Although these are present only in very small quantities, they may be smelled at concentrations as low as one part per million.

Some people resort to eating charcoal tablets to counteract any tendency to form smelly gas, but there is some doubt about their effectiveness in "absorbing" intestinal gas. You may help to alleviate your "gaseous" symptoms by changing your diet, especially reducing the amount of fiber if you normally have a high intake.

Borborygmi

This is the medical term for a noisy, gassy, gurgling abdomen. It may be a symptom of malabsorption or poor digestion, but occasionally it may be a sign of some kind of intestinal obstruction. However, when borborygmi is the main symptom and other diseases have been ruled out, the cause is almost always some kind of functional disturbance.

Bloating

Bloating affects women more than men. It may develop suddenly, sometimes after food, or it may come on gradually. It can make a woman look pregnant and in both sexes clothes feel tight. The swelling usually subsides within 24 hours.

It is caused by contraction of the diaphragm and the muscles in the lower back, which compresses the abdominal contents and pushes them forward. It often accompanies IBS and it is important to recognize that the condition is not caused by organic disease and no further investigation is required.

You don't need treatment unless it is very uncomfortable—and your doctor will simply explain why the problem occurs and reassure you. You may get some relief by lying flat and relaxing your muscles. If you're a very anxious person, your doctor may suggest some kind of treatment to help you relax (see page 91). Occasionally other medications are prescribed if the bloating is very bothersome.

Proctalgia fugax

Proctalgia fugax refers to a sudden pain felt deep in the rectum, which may last for a few seconds to several minutes and can vary in intensity. It usually happens at night and may or may not be associated with IBS, although it is not one of the standard features of the condition.

It is not serious in itself, and does not necessarily require treatment. If it is persistent and interferes with daily activities or sleep, a medication may sometimes be prescribed.

Trouble with initiating a bowel movement

People with IBS sometimes experience problems to do with starting a bowel movement. These can include:

- feeling no urge to defecate even though feces are present in the rectum
- painful involuntary straining (tenesmus)
- ineffectual and painful straining when trying to pass a stool
- the sensation that you can't completely empty your bowels.

Such difficulties are usually functional in origin, but your doctor will first want to perform a gentle rectal examination and possibly a sigmoidoscopy, to make sure that they are not caused by any organic disease.

KEY POINTS

■ A wide variety of gastrointestinal symptoms and disorders, originating from the mouth to the anus, are associated with IBS

■ Treatment for excessive anxiety can help to alleviate symptoms for many people

■ The intestines of people with IBS are particularly sensitive to gas

Treatment

A positive diagnosis can be reassuring
In the past, you would probably have been told you
had IBS only when all other possible causes for your
symptoms had been ruled out. Today it is diagnosed as
a condition in its own right based on the pattern of
symptoms and may not require further tests.

The fact that any tests have come back negative is
very reassuring. It is also reassuring to know that,
although your symptoms may be troublesome, they will
produce no complications whatsoever.

It is important to raise any worries you may have
such as fear of inflammation, ulceration, or cancer so
that your doctor can help put your mind at rest.

Psychological therapies
Many people with IBS also have underlying stress,
anxiety, or depression that makes their symptoms
worse. A number of psychological therapies can help,
although these are not always easily available.

What your doctor will do to help you

Once you have been diagnosed with IBS, your doctor will advise you of any changes that you need to make to reduce your symptoms. If there are any treatments that may help, your doctor will suggest these. Help includes the following:

- Reassurance that you do not have a serious illness such as cancer
- Treatment may be needed with bulk laxatives, anti-diarrheal, or anti-spasm medications
- Treatment may be needed for associated problems such as gynecological disorders
- Benefit may be obtained from an anti-anxiety or antidepressant drug treatment

Relaxation therapy

This is the simplest form of "psychotherapy" which you can easily learn from audiotapes. If stress is contributing to your IBS, then relaxation will help reduce your symptoms and give you a sense of well-being, so that you feel more confident and in control.

You will also be taught how to exclude sources of tension and to relax. Usually, around 10 sessions are needed.

Biofeedback

This depends on recognizing various signs of abnormal body function and learning how to correct them. It is most commonly used in the treatment of incontinence and constipation.

Therapy aims to make you more sensitive to rectal sensation and helps avoid excessive straining. It also provides a detailed explanation of how your body normally works, and helps retrain the muscles involved in having a bowel movement.

Hypnotherapy

Hypnosis is used to induce a state of relaxation and then to try to alter underlying abnormalities of gut motility and/or sensation.

The therapist will hypnotize you, with the ultimate aim of enabling you to control symptoms on your own, by making use of what you have learned during the treatment sessions. Success depends very much on the therapist being interested in treating IBS and these therapists are not widely available. Some people have success using self-hypnosis tapes designed for IBS treatment.

Cognitive–behavioral therapy

Cognitive–behavioral therapy (CBT) is based on the assumption that IBS in some people is related to the way you respond to what happens in your everyday life. CBT helps you recognize negative patterns of thinking and behavior.

It encourages you to change your interpretation of bodily sensations and functions by seeing them differently. It helps if you see them not so much as symptoms of disease that need to be treated, but more as expressions of stress or anxiety that are associated with particular life events. Treatment is essentially an exercise in identifying and solving problems, which allows you to gain a greater sense of control. These techniques have been repeatedly shown to be effective for IBS relief.

Dynamic psychotherapy

This helps to provide you with an insight into why particular symptoms have developed and what they might mean or represent in the light of changes in key relationships. These insights will help you make long-lasting changes in your normal attitudes and behavior patterns.

Symptoms often seem to stem from significant life changes (often the loss of a relationship) that are difficult to come to terms with. This therapy helps you work through relationship difficulties with the guidance of the therapist.

How effective are psychological therapies?

Most studies with behavioral therapy, psychotherapy, or hypnotherapy show that brief treatments result in a 60 to 70 percent improvement in IBS symptoms. This is better than the results of most medications for IBS. Young people who have had classic symptoms for a relatively short time do best. However, 15–20 percent of people with IBS do not benefit from psychological therapies.

Drug treatment

Unfortunately, most drug treatments for IBS are of only limited value and many have side effects. Nevertheless, some drugs may help certain symptoms in individual people.

It may be that you need only one drug, although some people do better on a combination of drugs. An example is a laxative or anti-diarrheal drug (see page 73) together with a drug that reduces muscle spasm or anxiety. A combination of an anti-anxiety drug and an antidepressant can relieve abdominal pain and diarrhea effectively for some people.

Combining drugs in this way may make it possible to control your condition with smaller doses than when one is prescribed on its own.

Anti-spasmodic drugs

If you suffer from pain caused by strong spasms in your colon, anti-spasmodic drugs may help. They act by relaxing the intestinal muscles.

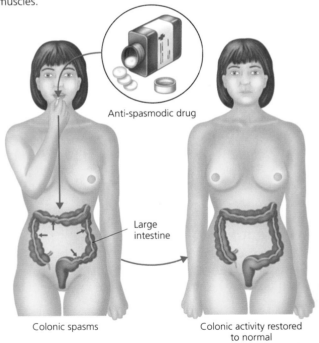

Anti-spasmodic drug

Large intestine

Colonic spasms

Colonic activity restored to normal

Anti-spasmodic drugs

Anti-spasmodic drugs (such as dicyclomine and hyoscyamine) relax intestinal smooth muscle. They may be helpful in relieving pain caused by spasms of the colon. Some people find that these drugs stop working after a while, but it is usually possible for your doctor to prescribe a related drug if this happens. This is likely to remain effective for a similar period of time to the first drug.

Antidepressant drugs

As well as treating underlying depression or anxiety, antidepressants can change the way that your gut muscles react and alter nerve responses from your gut. One family of drugs, called tricyclic antidepressants, slows down the rapid small bowel transit, which is the problem for people with diarrhea-predominant IBS. Another drug, called paroxetine (a selective serotonin reuptake inhibitor or SSRI), accelerates movement of the contents through the small bowel.

Both these treatments can relieve gut symptoms at doses too low to have any effect on your state of mind. Antidepressant medication has also been shown to have significant benefit in the treatment of pain. These drugs are most effective when taken at night.

Drugs that change bowel motility

These drugs affect the bowel response to serotonin. Serotonin (also known as hydroxytryptamine) is a hormone with an important role in the motor (movement) and secretory response of the gut to the ingestion of food. One of these drugs is alosetron which antagonizes type 3 serotonin (HT_3) receptors in the gut and is effective in diarrhea-predominant IBS, although rare vascular damage to the colon has been linked to its use. Due to its potentially dangerous side effects, it is usually only prescribed by a gastroenterologist.

Another is tegaserod, which stimulates type 4 serotonin (HT_4) receptors. It is used to treat constipation-predominant IBS and chronic constipation. It has also been shown to help bloating in some IBS patients.

Dietary treatment

If your diet is contributing to your symptoms, making changes can bring considerable relief. This could be something as simple as reducing your intake of natural fiber foods, fruit, or caffeine, if any are on the high side.

Some people, especially those of non-European descent, may not produce enough of the lactase enzyme (needed to digest the milk sugar, lactose). If you regularly consume more than half a pint of milk a day, you may benefit from cutting down.

A few people develop IBS symptoms from a high intake of fructose (fruit sugar) as a result of slow or incomplete absorption. It can cause gut distension to which people with IBS appear to be especially sensitive.

More often, people with IBS have symptoms due to eating, but there is no specific food or food group causing the problem. You may have already identified for yourself certain foods that trigger your symptoms, especially if you are prone to diarrhea. These trigger foods are different for everyone. If food-related symptoms lead you to limit the range of foods that you eat, you should ask your doctor to refer you to a dietitian to make sure that you continue to obtain all the nutrients that you need from your restricted diet.

Scientific evidence to support the theory that diets that avoid yeast-containing food or that are gluten-free will help cure IBS is lacking. Avoidance of yeast-containing foods has been suggested in the belief that this will prevent excessive growth of the *Candida* organism. Candida is a yeast-like organism that is normally present in the gut. However, scientific evidence suggests that Candida is not involved in causing IBS. A small minority of people find that excluding gluten (contained in wheat, barley, and rye) from their diet helps their IBS, but most stay the same or actually get worse.

Complementary and alternative therapies

A wide variety of complementary and alternative practices and therapies are commonly resorted to by IBS patients, both together with and instead of conventional treatment. As many of these therapies have never been subjected to controlled clinical trials, some of their efficacy may reflect a high placebo response rate.

There is, however, evidence to support the efficacy in IBS for some forms of herbal therapy and certain probiotics.

Probiotics are "friendly bacteria," such as Lactobacillus and Bifidus bacteria. They have several actions that may be of benefit in IBS. These include antibacterial effects, protection of the gut lining, and influencing immune reactions in the gut. More information is needed before probiotics can be recommended to all people with IBS, such as which specific types are most beneficial, in what doses, and for which symptoms should they be taken.

Chinese herbal therapy has been effective for some people with IBS but requires a specialist trained in oriental medicine to determine the correct combination of herbs, and the long-term safety of these herbs is not known. Peppermint oil supplements have also been used for IBS pain and bloating, though they may have side effects and don't appear to help bowel movement problems. Aloe vera is a herbal remedy that has been used medically for thousands of years. Some people claim that it has helped their symptoms of IBS. Others, however, have reported that their symptoms have worsened with the use of aloe vera. In the absence of properly conducted clinical trials showing any benefit, its routine use cannot be recommended.

Acupuncture is used by some people with IBS, but current clinical trials show that it is no better than a placebo.

When treatment doesn't help

Around five percent of people continue to experience abdominal pain that causes a major disturbance to their lives, despite having tried all the standard treatments. This can be frustrating for both doctor and patient, especially when investigations repeatedly find no cause for the problem.

It might seem logical for the person to seek out second or even third opinions from other doctors. In practice this often doesn't help, however, and can just make the existing anxiety worse, quite apart from the expense.

A more successful approach may be for you to continue to see the same doctor (either your general physician or a gastroenterologist) every few months, to review the situation and discuss your current symptoms. Eventually, this may help you find solutions for your IBS and enhance your ability to cope with it.

KEY POINTS

- The diagnosis of IBS is a positive one, and is not based simply on ruling out any other possible causes for your symptoms

- Don't be upset if your doctor suggests that psychological issues may have a role in either causing or increasing your symptoms, as this is often the case

- Psychological therapies, including relaxation therapy, biofeedback, hypnotherapy, and psychotherapy, are often helpful

- Drug treatments for IBS don't work for everyone, but may help to relieve individual symptoms

- Sometimes a change in your diet may relieve symptoms if diet is helping trigger your symptoms

What happens now?

Living with IBS

If you are seeing your general internist, or have been referred to a specialist, whether you need further appointments and, if so, how frequently will depend on your personal situation. You may well have found that you have been given a satisfactory explanation for your symptoms and don't need to see the doctor again, especially if your IBS is no more than a minor inconvenience. Other people do best by having several monthly appointments until their symptoms start to improve.

You may need to have follow-up appointments if you have been advised to alter your diet and/or if you have been put on medication. This is so that your response to treatment can be assessed.

However, it is important that you have a good line of communication with either your general doctor or gastroenterologist so that you feel that you can return if you need to. Some people will need to continue seeing their doctor on a regular basis, to monitor the situation and discuss symptoms and worries.

If you think your doctor is unsympathetic and you cannot establish a good relationship with him or her, you may want to find a doctor with a particular interest in IBS.

Outlook

Unfortunately, once a person has contracted IBS, they are prone to recurrent symptoms. Some have long periods of relief between IBS flareups; others have persistent symptoms that wax and wane with time.

A substantial proportion of individuals with IBS become free from symptoms over a 12-month period, but may develop other functional symptoms such as indigestion (dyspepsia) in their place. One study found that around 30 percent of people with IBS still had symptoms after five years. Another study found that only five percent of people were completely symptom-free after five years.

You are likely to have a less optimistic outlook in terms of getting rid of your symptoms if:

- psychological factors (such as anxiety) play a major role in causing them
- you have had IBS for a long time
- you have had abdominal surgery.

Most people learn to live with IBS and find that explanation and reassurance from their doctor are the most important aspect of their treatment. You should always let your doctor know if your symptoms change significantly. However, once the diagnosis of IBS is established, the chances of developing some new and serious disease are extremely low.

KEY POINTS

■ IBS is a long-term problem so, although symptoms may come and go, a permanent cure is unlikely

■ Whether you need to have follow-up appointments once your condition has been diagnosed will depend on individual circumstances

■ Most people can learn to live with their IBS symptoms which, although they can be troublesome, are unlikely to lead to complications

■ If you have been diagnosed with IBS, the diagnosis is unlikely to change in the future

Useful organizations

Where can I find out more?

We have included the following organizations because, on preliminary investigation, they may be of use to the reader. However, we do not have first-hand experience of every organization and so cannot guarantee the organization's integrity. The reader must therefore exercise his or her own discretion and judgment when making further enquiries.

Canadian Society of Intestinal Research
855 West 12th Avenue
Vancouver, British Columbia
Canada V5Z 1M9
Phone: 604–875–4875
Fax: 604–875–4429
Website: www.badgut.com

This charitable foundation provides information on a wide variety of gastrointestinal disorders, including IBS.

IBS Self Help Group (Irritable Bowel Syndrome Association)
1440 Whalley Avenue, No. 145,
New Haven CT 06515
Email: ibsa@ibsassociation.org
Website: www.ibsassociation.org

U.S.-based international website with information and online forum; provides access to bulletin boards and forums, book list and store, medication and clinical study listings. No implied endorsement of sponsored products advertised; all donations fund activities of the Group.

International Foundation for Functional Gastrointestinal Disorders (IFFGD)
P.O. Box 170864
Milwaukee, WI 53217–8076
Phone 1–414–964–1799
Fax 1–414–964–7176
Website: www.iffgd.org

A nonprofit education and research organization. Comprehensive website for IBS patients. Multiple publications and links.

National Health Information Center (NHIC)
Online: www.health.gov/NHIC
PO Box 1133
Washington, DC 20013
Tel: (800) 336–4797

NHIC, part of the Department of Health and Human Services, helps people locate information on health issues through referral to organizations that can best answer their questions.

National Institute of Diabetes and Digestive and Kidney Diseases (NIDDK)
NIDDK Clearinghouses Publications Catalog
5 Information Way
Bethesda, MD 20892–3568
Website: www.niddk.nih.gov

This division of the National Institutes of Health provides health education information for a wide array of gastrointestinal illnesses, including IBS. Healthcare education publications are available through the NIDDK Clearinghouse.

UCLA Center for Neurovisceral Sciences and Women's Health
GLAVAHS, Building 115/CURE, Room 222A
11301 Wilshire Blvd
Los Angeles, CA 90073
Website: www.cns.med.ucla.edu

The Center is focused on research involving IBS and other functional disorders to find a better understanding of the underlying causes and to develop new treatments. The mind-brain-body interaction and effect of sex in development of these disorders is emphasized. The website has an educational section for patients as well as a listing of current research studies recruiting patients.

University of North Carolina Center for Functional GI and Motility Disorders
CB#7080, Bioinformatics Building
Chapel Hill, NC 27599–7080
Website: www.med.unc.edu/medicine/fgidc/

This University Center provides a wide array of patient education materials and information about patient care and research on its website. The Center focuses on gastrointestinal motility.

www.ClinicalTrials.gov
This site was developed by the U.S. National Institutes of Health to provide information about current research studies recruiting patients.

The internet as a source of further information

After reading this book, you may feel that you would like further information on the subject. The internet is, of course, an excellent place to look and there are many websites with useful information about medical disorders, related charities, and support groups.

For those who do not have a computer at home, some cafés offer facilities for accessing the internet. Your local library offers a similar facility and has staff to help you find the information that you need.

It should always be remembered, however, that the internet is unregulated and anyone is free to set up a website and add information to it. Many websites offer impartial advice and information that has been compiled and checked by qualified medical professionals. Some, on the other hand, are run by commercial organizations for the purpose of promoting their own products. Others still are run by independent groups, some of which may be suggesting medications or treatments that are not supported by the medical and scientific community.

Always remember the internet is international and unregulated. It holds a wealth of valuable information but individual sites may be biased, out-of-date—or just plain wrong. The publisher accepts no responsibility for the content of links published in this series.

Index

Your pages

We have included the following pages because they may help you manage your illness or condition and its treatment.

Before an appointment with a health professional, it can be useful to write down a short list of questions of things that you do not understand, so that you can make sure that you do not forget anything.

Some of the sections may not be relevant to your circumstances.

Thank you

Health-care contact details

Name:

Practitioner type:

Place of work:

Tel:

Name:

Practitioner type:

Place of work:

Tel:

Name:

Practitioner type:

Place of work:

Tel:

Name:

Practitioner type:

Place of work:

Tel:

Significant past health events—illnesses/operations/investigations/treatments

Event	Month	Year	Age (at time)

Appointments for health care

Name:

Place:

Date:

Time:

Tel:

Name:

Place:

Date:

Time:

Tel:

Name:

Place:

Date:

Time:

Tel:

Name:

Place:

Date:

Time:

Tel:

Appointments for health care

Name:

Place:

Date:

Time:

Tel:

Name:

Place:

Date:

Time:

Tel:

Name:

Place:

Date:

Time:

Tel:

Name:

Place:

Date:

Time:

Tel:

Current medication(s) prescribed by your doctor

Medicine name:

Purpose:

Frequency & dose:

Start date:

End date:

Medicine name:

Purpose:

Frequency & dose:

Start date:

End date:

Medicine name:

Purpose:

Frequency & dose:

Start date:

End date:

Medicine name:

Purpose:

Frequency & dose:

Start date:

End date:

Other medicines/supplements you are taking, not prescribed by your doctor

Medicine/treatment:

Purpose:

Frequency & dose:

Start date:

End date:

Medicine/treatment:

Purpose:

Frequency & dose:

Start date:

End date:

Medicine/treatment:

Purpose:

Frequency & dose:

Start date:

End date:

Medicine/treatment:

Purpose:

Frequency & dose:

Start date:

End date:

Questions to ask at appointments
(Note: do bear in mind that doctors work under great time pressure, so long lists may not be helpful for either of you)

Questions to ask at appointments
(Note: do bear in mind that doctors work under great time pressure, so long lists may not be helpful for either of you)

Notes

Notes

Notes

Notes

Notes

Notes

Notes

Notes

Notes

Notes

Notes

Notes

Notes

Notes

Notes